PCOS DIET

A Beginner's Guide to Reverse PCOS, Repair Your Metabolism and Restore Fertility

Clair Simeon

TABLE OF CONTENT

TABLE OF CONTENTS

CHAPTER 1

Introduction to PCOS and Fertility

PCOS, also known as polycystic ovary syndrome, is a prevalent hormonal condition that can affect up to 20% of women who are of reproductive age. It is defined by an imbalance of hormones such as estrogen and testosterone, as well as the appearance of small fluid-filled sacs (cysts) on the ovaries. Additionally, it is characterized by the presence of fluid-filled cysts on the ovaries.

PCOS can result in a wide variety of symptoms, some of which include acne, trouble conceiving a child, infrequent or nonexistent periods, and excessive hair growth on the face and body. Additionally, it is related with an increased risk of certain health disorders, such as insulin resistance, type 2 diabetes, and cardiovascular disease.

PCOS is characterized by hormonal imbalances and irregular ovulation, both of which can have a negative impact on a woman's fertility. This is often the case in women who suffer from this disorder. It is essential to keep in mind, however, that even women who have PCOS have the potential to conceive a child if they receive the appropriate medical care and emotional support.

PCOS is a condition that currently has no known therapy or cure, but it can be controlled by a variety of methods, including adjustments to one's lifestyle, medicine, and other approaches. Diet and nutrition are two of the most important aspects of PCOS management since eating the appropriate meals and getting the right nutrients can help restore hormonal balance and boost fertility. This book will discuss the correlation between polycystic ovary syndrome (PCOS) and infertility, as well as offer a comprehensive strategy for treating the illness by modifying one's food and way of life. Therefore, this book provides a comprehensive guide to improving a woman's reproductive health and raising the likelihood that she will become pregnant in cases when she has PCOS.

CHAPTER 2

The Link Between Diet and Fertility

In women who suffer from polycystic ovary syndrome (PCOS), the foods they consume can have a major influence on their ability to conceive. In point of fact, a number of studies have demonstrated that modifying one's diet in a certain way can assist in restoring hormone balance, normalizing menstrual cycles, and elevating a woman's fertility in cases of polycystic ovary syndrome (PCOS).

Maintaining tight control over your blood sugar levels is an essential component of a PCOS diet designed to boost fertility. Insulin resistance, which can alter hormone balance and interfere with ovulation, is more likely to occur in women who have polycystic ovary syndrome (PCOS). You can assist in the regulation of blood sugar levels and improve insulin sensitivity by consuming a diet that is low in refined carbohydrates and high in fiber, protein, and healthy fats.

It is essential to place an emphasis, in addition to managing blood sugar levels, on obtaining a wide range of nutrients from meals that are whole and unprocessed. This includes consuming an adequate amount of healthy fats, such as omega-3 fatty acids, which can assist in the reduction of inflammation and the improvement of hormone balance. The consumption of an adequate amount of antioxidants, such as those that are present in fruits and vegetables, may also be advantageous for fertility.

When attempting to follow a diet that is meant to boost fertility in PCOS patients, it is essential to pay attention to portion sizes as well as calorie intake. It is possible that some women who have PCOS will need to reduce their body mass in order to restore hormone balance and boost their chances of becoming pregnant. On the other hand, having a low body mass index can interfere with menstrual periods as well as fertility. It may be important to work with a healthcare physician or a qualified dietitian in order to determine the appropriate calorie intake and the appropriate balance of macronutrients for your needs.

Alterations to one's diet and way of life, as well as other aspects of one's lifestyle, will be the focus of the following chapter, in which we will examine a holistic approach to the management of PCOS and the enhancement of fertility.

CHAPTER 3

A Holistic Approach to Managing PCOS

It is not enough to simply treat the hormonal imbalances and symptoms of PCOS in order to be successful in managing the illness. It is essential to take a comprehensive approach to one's health that addresses all areas of one's wellbeing, such as one's diet, physical activity, and ability to cope with stress.

PCOS can be effectively managed, and fertility can be improved, with proper nutrition. You can help balance hormone levels and increase insulin sensitivity by following a diet designed specifically for people with polycystic ovary syndrome (PCOS). This diet should be high in foods that are whole and unprocessed and low in refined carbohydrates and added sugars. Because weight management can be a factor in increasing fertility in people with PCOS, it is also very important to pay attention to the sizes of the portions that you eat and the calories that you consume.

In addition to proper nutrition, engaging in regular physical activity can assist in restoring hormone balance, normalizing menstrual cycles, and enhancing a woman's ability to become pregnant in cases of polycystic ovary syndrome (PCOS). Aim for at least 150 minutes of activity per week at a moderate intensity, or for at least 75 minutes of exercise per week at a strong intensity. Incorporating strength training and flexibility workouts into your program is also something that should not be overlooked.

The control of stress is another crucial component in the process of treating PCOS and achieving optimal fertility. Long-term stress can throw off the natural balance of hormones and prevent ovulation from occurring. It is possible to enhance your general health and boost the likelihood of becoming pregnant by incorporating stress-relieving activities like meditation, yoga, or deep breathing into your daily routine.

In the following chapter, we will delve into the intricacies of the PCOS-specific nutrition plan and provide step-by-step guidance on the appropriate foods and nutrients to support fertility and manage PCOS symptoms. In addition, we will discuss the PCOS-specific nutrition plan in further detail.

CHAPTER 4

The PCOS-Specific Nutrition Plan

Finding the correct meals and nutrients can make a significant impact on both the management of PCOS and the improvement of fertility. In this chapter, we will present a step-by-step guide to the dietary plan that is particular to PCOS. This guide will include the sorts of foods that should be prioritized as well as those that should be limited or avoided.

Focusing on whole, unprocessed foods that are high in nutrients but low in added sugars and refined carbohydrates is the first and most crucial step toward improving one's diet. This entails eating a lot of vegetables, fruits, and whole grains, as well as lean protein sources like chicken, fish, and plant-based alternatives.

In addition to these essentials, there are a number of essential nutrients that have been shown to be especially helpful in the management of PCOS and the enhancement of fertility. These are the following:

Fiber: Aim for at least 25-30 grams of fiber each day to help manage blood sugar and enhance insulin sensitivity. Fiber can be found in whole grains, vegetables, and fruits. Vegetables, fruits, whole grains, and legumes are all excellent food choices that are high in fiber.

Include in your diet foods that are sources of healthy fats, such as olive oil, avocados, almonds, and seeds, to assist in the reduction of inflammation and the improvement of hormone balance.

Antioxidants: Getting a sufficient amount of antioxidants in one's diet might help boost one's fertility as well as their general health. Fruits and vegetables, particularly those with a vivid coloration like berries, leafy greens, and sweet potatoes, are excellent sources. Other good sources include nuts and seeds.

On the other hand, if you are following a diet designed specifically for PCOS, there are certain categories of foods and nutrients that you should try to limit or avoid altogether. These are the following:

These foods can cause a surge in blood sugar and contribute to insulin resistance, both of which can be factors in PCOS and fertility. Refined carbohydrates and added sugars are also potentially problematic. Reduce your consumption of refined carbohydrates, such as white bread, spaghetti, and pastries, and opt instead for whole grains. Sugars that are added to foods should be avoided as much as possible; this includes the sugars that are found in sweetened beverages and processed snacks.

These harmful lipids, known as trans fats, are known to exacerbate inflammation and contribute to insulin resistance. Stay away from foods that contain trans fats or partially hydrogenated oils, as well as any additional sources of trans fats.

You may help improve the hormone balance and boost your chances of getting pregnant even if you have PCOS by include these nutrient-rich, whole foods in your diet and restricting or avoiding others that may be less effective. In the following chapter, we are going to make it as simple as possible for you to adhere to the PCOS-specific dietary plan by providing meal planning and dish ideas.

CHAPTER 5

Meal Planning and Recipe Ideas
for the PCOS Fertility Diet

If you have polycystic ovary syndrome (PCOS), following a diet designed for that condition can help improve hormone balance, control menstrual cycles, and enhance the likelihood of becoming pregnant. On the other hand, it isn't always easy to figure out what you should be eating on a regular basis. In this chapter, we will make it simple for you to adhere to the PCOS fertility diet by providing sample meal plans and suggestions for recipes.

First things first, let's get familiar with the fundamentals of meal planning. Aim to fill each meal and snack with a range of wholesome foods that are high in various nutrients. This should include a large quantity of vegetables, fruits, cereals that are whole, and sources of lean protein. Because weight management can be a factor in increasing fertility in people with PCOS, it is also very important to pay attention to the sizes of the portions that you eat and the calories that you consume.

The following is a list of some general advice to bear in mind when planning meals:

develop a shopping list: After you have planned out your meals and snacks for the week, develop a shopping list of the ingredients that you will need to purchase at the store. This can help you keep organized and prevent you from making hasty purchases of items that are less nutritious.

Plan ahead: Pick a day of the week to perform some meal

preparation, such as chopping vegetables, cooking grains, or preparing sources of protein. For example, you could cut vegetables, cook grains, or prepare sources of protein. This might be a time saver and make it easier to adhere to the reproductive diet for PCOS during the week.

Maintain a supply of healthy snacks: Keeping a supply of healthy snacks such as nuts, seeds, veggies, and fruit on hand will help prevent feelings of hunger as well as cravings for foods that are less healthy.

Now that we've covered the general principles of the PCOS fertility diet, let's talk about some specific dish ideas. In addition to being simple to put together, the meals and snacks that are included here are loaded with the nutrients that can assist in restoring hormone balance and increasing fertility.

For breakfast, you might want to try a bowl of oats topped with chopped nuts, berries, and honey drizzle. Alternately, you may prepare an omelette with spinach, mushrooms, and whole grain bread.

For lunch, pack a salad consisting of quinoa, black beans, plenty of vegetables, and a vinaigrette that you made yourself. You may also try a wrap made of turkey, avocado, and whole grain bread.

Prepare a stir-fry with a large quantity of vegetables and the protein of your choosing, and serve it atop brown rice for dinner. You might also try fish that has been grilled and served with roasted veggies and quinoa.

Snacks: If you're hungry between meals, grab a handful of nuts, a piece of fruit, or make yourself a homemade smoothie with some yogurt, fruit, and spinach.

You may simply adhere to the PCOS fertility diet by including these nutritious and delectable meal and snack options into your daily routine. In doing so, you will take a step toward boosting both

your fertility and your general
health.

CHAPTER 6

Addressing Other Factors that Can Impact Fertility with PCOS

In addition to dietary choices, there are a number of other aspects of a woman's lifestyle that can have an effect on her fertility if she has PCOS. In this chapter, we will discuss many ways in which one might improve their reproductive health by making adjustments to their food and lifestyle.

Management of stress is an important factor to take into consideration. Because chronic stress can alter hormone balance and interfere with ovulation, it can make it more challenging for a couple to conceive a child. It is possible to enhance your general health and boost the likelihood of becoming pregnant by incorporating stress-relieving activities like meditation, yoga, or deep breathing into your daily routine.

The importance of physical activity cannot be overstated. In women who have polycystic ovary syndrome (PCOS), engaging in regular physical activity can assist improve hormone balance, control menstrual cycles, and enhance the likelihood that they will become pregnant.

Aim for at least 150 minutes of activity per week at a moderate intensity, or for at least 75 minutes of exercise per week at a strong intensity. Incorporating strength training and flexibility workouts into your program is also something that should not be overlooked.

In addition to getting enough exercise and learning how to better handle stress, paying attention to the quality and quantity of sleep you get is quite important. A sufficient amount of sleep is necessary for maintaining general health and can also assist in the regulation of hormone levels and the improvement of fertility. Aim to get between 7 and 9 hours of sleep each night.

Other aspects of one's way of life that should be taken into account include avoiding tobacco and alcohol and cutting down on one's exposure to environmental contaminants. These can throw off the natural balance of hormones and cause problems with fertility.

Last but not least, it is essential to consult a healthcare professional or fertility specialist in order to establish the treatment strategy that is most appropriate for your specific requirements. This may include the use of hormone-balancing drugs and other fertility treatments, such as in vitro fertilization (IVF), as well as the possibility of taking medication to improve fertility.

You may take a comprehensive approach to maximizing your fertility and increasing your chances of getting pregnant even if you have PCOS by addressing five critical lifestyle factors in addition to following a diet designed specifically for women with PCOS.

CHAPTER 7

Supplementation and Natural Remedies for PCOS and Fertility

Alterations to one's diet and way of life are not the only things that can help manage PCOS and improve fertility; certain supplements and natural therapies may also be beneficial. However, it is essential to emphasize that these options should only be pursued in conjunction with standard medical therapy and under the supervision of a qualified medical professional. They should in no way be considered alternatives to standard medical care.

Omega-3 fatty acids are one type of supplement that some women who have PCOS have found to be helpful. Inflammation can be reduced and hormone balance can be improved with the help of these beneficial fats. Either you eat foods that naturally contain them, including fatty fish, nuts, and seeds, or you can take a supplement of them.

Chromium is yet another dietary supplement that has been demonstrated to be useful in restoring normal hormone levels and insulin sensitivity in PCOS patients who are female. This trace mineral can be obtained from foods like whole grains, nuts, and vegetables, or it can be taken as a supplement. Both options are available.

PCOS can be managed and fertility can be improved with the use of supplements, but there are also natural therapies and herbs that may be of assistance. These are the following:

Vitex agnus-castus, often known as chasteberry, is a herb that has been demonstrated to boost fertility in women who suffer from PCOS and assist control their menstrual cycles.

Green tea: The polyphenols and other antioxidants found in green tea have been shown to have positive effects on insulin sensitivity and inflammation in women with PCOS.

It has been demonstrated that cinnamon can enhance insulin sensitivity and lower blood sugar levels in women who suffer from PCOS.

Before beginning use of any new supplement or natural cure, it is always ideal to talk with a healthcare provider or a certified practitioner. It is crucial to keep in mind that the safety and effectiveness of natural remedies might vary, and it is always preferable to make this point clear.

In the following chapter, we will go over some effective methods for overcoming typical obstacles that arise when adhering to a PCOS-specific diet and maximizing fertility by making adjustments to one's lifestyle.

CHAPTER 8

**Overcoming Common
Challenges When Following the
PCOS Fertility Diet**

It can be tough to make adjustments to your food and lifestyle, particularly if you have been accustomed to certain routines for a significant amount of time. However, it is possible to stick to the PCOS fertility diet and experience favorable effects in terms of hormone balance and fertility if the appropriate tactics and support are utilized.

Cravings for foods that are less healthful are a common obstacle faced by people who are trying to follow a new diet. It is perfectly normal to have desires for specific meals; however, it is essential to put in place measures that will assist you in managing these cravings and staying on track with your goals. The following are some ways that can be used to manage cravings:

Organize your meals and snacks for the week, as well as compile a shopping list, by making preparations in advance. This can be helpful in preventing impulsive purchasing of items that are less healthful.

Keeping nutritious food and drink alternatives on hand: Maintaining a ready supply of nutritious snacks, such as nuts, seeds, veggies, and fruit, will assist in warding off cravings and ensuring that you remain content.

Treating yourself occasionally is acceptable as long as you keep track of the calories and nutrients you consume and ensure that your occasional indulgence does not throw off your overall calorie and nutrient intake. You should make an effort to choose out sweets that include fewer added sugars and refined carbohydrates.

When trying to follow a diet for PCOS fertility, one of the main challenges that people have is the feeling of being overwhelmed or unclear of what to eat. Working with a registered dietitian or a healthcare provider to develop an individualized meal plan that caters to your specific requirements and objectives can be of great assistance in this endeavor. In addition, there is a wealth of information pertaining to meal planning and recipe creation that can be found both online and in printed cookbooks.

When making modifications to your lifestyle and diet, it is essential to surround yourself with people who will encourage you and hold you accountable. Support can come from a variety of sources, such as friends and family, a healthcare provider, or a support group. When trying to conceive a child with PCOS, it might be helpful to have someone to talk to and share your experiences with in order to make the effort of adhering to a PCOS fertility diet feel more bearable.

You can overcome typical hurdles and successfully follow the PCOS fertility diet to improve hormone balance and increase the likelihood of becoming pregnant if you take proactive measures and seek support when you feel you need it.

CHAPTER **9**

Supporting Your Fertility Journey

It may be a journey that demands patience, persistence, and a willingness to make adjustments in order to successfully manage PCOS and optimize fertility through changes in food and lifestyle. It is essential to keep in mind that the experience of PCOS and fertility is different for every woman, and that treatments that are successful for one individual may not be effective for another.

In addition to this, it is essential to have reasonable expectations and to be well-prepared for any potential obstacles that may arise along the route. It is possible that seeing gains in hormone balance and fertility may take some time, and there is also a possibility that there may be fluctuations along the road. Even if you are making sluggish progress toward your objectives, it is essential to maintain patience and to keep moving in the right direction.

In addition to displaying patience and perseverance, it is essential to be nice to oneself and to keep in mind that it is OK to solicit assistance when it is required.

It might be beneficial to have a support system in place, whether it consists of friends, family, a healthcare provider, or a support group. Having this in place can be useful.

Last but not least, keep in mind that there are a lot of different approaches you may take to treat PCOS and increase your chances of getting pregnant. Alterations to one's food and way of life aren't the only things that can help improve fertility and regulate hormone levels; there are also drugs and other types of therapies that can be helpful. It is essential to collaborate with a healthcare professional or fertility specialist in order to select the treatment plan that is most appropriate for your specific requirements.

You can improve your chances of becoming pregnant and reduce the severity of PCOS by taking a holistic approach to treating your condition and maximizing your fertility, as well as by seeking support when you feel you need it.